A Patient's and Clii

Saving
Your Teeth,
Your Implants
And
Your Health

Thomas K. McCawley, D.D.S., F.A.C.D.
Mark N. McCawley, D.M.D., M.S.

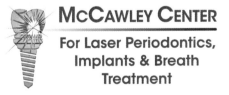

McCawley Center
For Laser Periodontics,
Implants & Breath
Treatment

Established 1972
"Saving Lives by Saving Smiles"

5th Edition

ISBN 978-0-9855111-2-8

5th Edition 2024

Table of Contents

Acknowledgements

This book would not have been possible without the incredible support and advice of our wife and mother, Brenda McCawley, and Ann Nye West, our brilliant editor and publisher. They were both amazingly patient with our numerous rewrites and additions.

Thanks also goes to our mentors, Drs. Jerry Kramer, Paul Keyes, Jorgen Slots and Tom Rams. They taught us the importance of identifying and treating the specific bacterial causes of periodontal disease which we discuss throughout the book.

Our patients, referring dentists, and team members also helped and inspired us by their questions and their advice about how best to save smiles for a lifetime.

Drs. Tom and Mark McCawley

Introduction
The Purpose of This Guide

Almost 50 percent of the people in the United States have gum disease, and about 30 million wear dentures primarily because of it. In addition, gum disease affects your overall health. It increases the risk of heart attacks, stroke, pancreatic cancer, Alzheimer's disease and many other serious systemic diseases.

With this in mind, the purpose of this guide is to assist patients, clinicians and team members in understanding periodontal disease and dental implants to better achieve our practice mission for our patients, "Saving Lives by Saving Smiles."

Our goal is to offer our patients therapies that we would want for ourselves. We have literally searched the world for the most gentle and effective treatments.

This has led us to minimally-invasive treatments that combine accurate diagnosis of the causes of periodontal and implant infections with proven laser, antibiotic, antiseptic and implant therapies to provide predictable, long-lasting treatment to save lives...and smiles.

For questions not answered in this book, please feel free to call us at the office at 954-522-3228 or email us at info@mccawley.com. More information, including videos with more extensive answers to many of the questions in the book, is also available by visiting our website, mccawley. com.

Yours in Better Total Health,
Drs. Tom and Mark McCawley

Summary:
What Causes Periodontal Disease
And How Is It Best Treated?

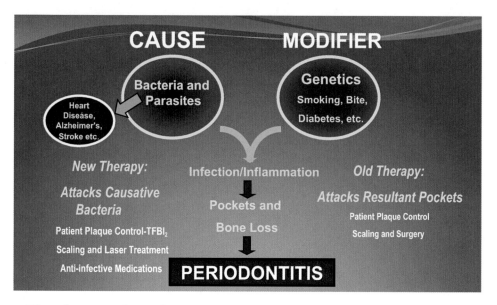

This diagram shows how bacteria and parasites, modified by genetics, viruses, and other factors, combine to cause infection and inflammation. This process in turn results in pockets and bone loss – periodontitis. Our practice focuses on treating the bacterial and parasitic cause of periodontal disease, not just the resultant pockets. We use special patient plaque control methods, proven laser treatments, and targeted anti-infective medications. This is the best way to control and/or eliminate the periodontal infection, and save your smile.

These therapies may also save your health. The bacteria and parasites which cause periodontal disease contribute to an increased incidence of heart disease, Alzheimer's disease, stroke, rheumatoid arthritis, pancreatic cancer, and many other systemic diseases.

Periodontal Disease
And Tooth Loss

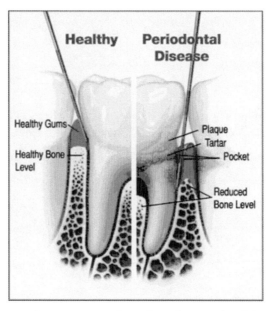

This illustration shows a periodontal probe in a healthy 3mm sulcus on the left, and in a diseased 6mm pocket showing bone loss on the right.

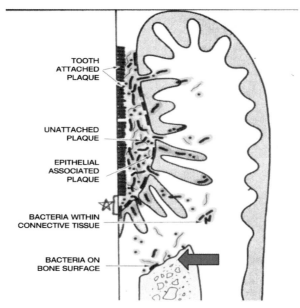

This illustration shows a periodontal pocket infected by millions of pathogenic bacteria and parasites that are eating away at the bone supporting the tooth. The bacteria and parasites then invade the adjacent gum tissue, allowing them to enter the bloodstream, spread throughout the body, and affect your health.

What Is Periodontal Disease?

I f your fingernails bled when you washed them, you would be concerned. Bleeding gums always indicate disease. Yet, many people think it's normal if their gums bleed when they brush or floss.

In a 1999 study, researchers at the U.S. National Institutes of Health (NIH) found that half of Americans over the age of 30 had bleeding gums. Recent studies have reported that almost 50 percent of the population in the United States has some form of periodontal disease. The disease is usually painless so we often don't know we have it until very late.

Swollen and bleeding gums are early signs that your gums are infected with bacteria and parasites. If nothing is done, the infection can spread and destroy the structures that support your teeth in your jawbone and affect your health. (See Summary of What Causes Periodontal Disease on page 6.)

Eventually, your teeth can become so loose that they have to be extracted. Other signs of periodontal disease include bad breath, gums that have receded from the tooth, loose or separated teeth, and pus when you press on the gums.

"Perio" means around, and "dontal" refers to teeth. Periodontal diseases are infections of the structures around the teeth, which include the gums, the periodontal ligament (which holds the teeth in), and alveolar bone.

In the earliest stage of periodontal disease – gingivitis – the infection affects the gums. In more severe forms of the disease – periodontitis – all of the tissues, including the supporting bone of the teeth, are involved. (See illustrations on the previous page.)

Peri-implantitis refers to the same periodontal disease occurring around implants.

Periodontal disease is a serious infection that does not go away on its own, nor get better with time. Prompt treatment is essential to save your teeth and implants and preserve your health. **Neglecting treatment is ultimately more expensive.**

Are you infected?

		Oral Flora
Healthy	• The gums are pink. • The edge of the gum adheres to the teeth. • No bleeding.	• Coccoid Bacteria • <u>Nonmotile</u> filamentous bacteria
Gingivitis	• The gums bleed easily. • Bad breath and a bad taste in the mouth occur. • The gums are reddish in color.	• <u>Motile</u> curved-shaped rods
Early Periodontitis	• Gums recede. • Bleeding is more pronounced. • Radiography shows a slight bone deterioration. • A **4 mm** pocket appears around the teeth.	• <u>White blood cells</u> • Motile spiral-shaped bacteria
Moderate Periodontitis	• Abscesses can develop around the teeth. Gums recede. • Radiography shows angular bone deterioration. • The pockets reach **5-6 mm**.	• <u>Pus formation</u> • Motile bacteria • Amoeba parasites
Advanced Periodontitis	• Teeth begin to loosen. • The pockets now reach **7+ mm**. The bone shows significant deterioration.	• Pus formation • Motile bacteria • <u>Nests of parasites</u>

How Will I Know if
I Have Gum Disease?

There are several signs that indicate gum disease: red, swollen or bleeding gums. Look closely in the mirror. If your gums look red or swollen, it's gum disease. (See previous page for signs of gum disease.)

If there is bleeding while brushing, flossing, or eating hard foods, it's gum disease. **Bleeding always indicates gum disease!**

Loose or shifting teeth usually indicates that bone loss is occurring from gum disease.

Bad breath from the bacteria or pus beneath the gum indicates gum disease.

And, finally, receding gums – getting "longer in the tooth" – is an indication of gum disease.

It is important to identify gum disease early before it becomes serious. Treatment of advanced disease is difficult, if not impossible.

About 30 million people in the United States have lost all of their teeth, mostly as a result of periodontal disease. As a result, they must wear dentures that cause poor chewing, premature aging, and health risks.

Your dentist, hygienist, or periodontist can determine if you have gum disease by measuring the depth of the pockets around your teeth with an instrument called a periodontal probe. (See illustration on page 8.)

What Is a Periodontist?

In brief, a dentist who has spent three extra years after dental school learning how to diagnose and treat periodontal diseases and place implants can call himself or herself a periodontist.

To begin with, students must first obtain an undergraduate degree from a college or university. They then apply for dental school, and are admitted if their grades and scores are exceptional. Only about one out of ten applicants are admitted. They then spend four years in dental school and earn a doctor of dental surgery (D.D.S.) or doctor of dental medicine (D.M.D.) degree. Both degrees are identical.

Next, those with an interest apply to highly competitive periodontal graduate programs. They spend an additional three years learning how to treat periodontal disease and place implants, and receive a postgraduate certificate that certifies them as periodontal specialists.

> *"I don't think I could ever put into words how THANKFUL I am for my periodontists, Dr. Thomas McCawley, Dr. Mark McCawley and their incredible staff.*
> *"I was so fortunate to have such a dedicated team of professionals there for my well-being during the year and a half process that without question has restored my life back to a healthy and happy one full of endless smiles!"*
> *Donna Barnes, Williston, North Dakota*

What Should I Look for In a Periodontal Examination?

1. Does the examination take more than one hour? Does the clinician listen to my questions and concerns and review my medical and dental history with me first, and then do a comprehensive oral examination?

2. Does the examination include an oral cancer screening, an evaluation of bite forces that may aggravate gum problems, a joint and muscle assessment, an evaluation of pockets, recession, bleeding, breath and pus, how loose the teeth are, and a complimentary 3D CBCT scan?

3. Does it note tooth decay and defective crowns and fillings?

4. Most importantly, are the causative bacteria evaluated on a phase contrast microscope for the presence of pathogenic bacteria and protozoa-like amoeba? If indicated for more advanced disease, a bacterial culture should be taken and sent to a laboratory for analysis.

5. Are low radiation digital radiographs taken and studied if they are not available from the referring office?

6. Does the clinician review the findings with me and explain the recommended treatment in detail, focusing on minimally-invasive treatments, using a laser for pockets and infection, and Pinhole Surgery for receded gums? Does the clinician consult with my restorative dentist and outline any restorative care that is needed?

7. Finally, does the office offer payment options to make the treatment more affordable.

"My examination appointment was made immediately, performed thoroughly, the procedures done successfully, and followed up impeccably by an exemplary staff with a superb knowledge of dentistry."

Anita Kellerman, Plantation, FL
5 out of 5 stars

What are the treatment choices?

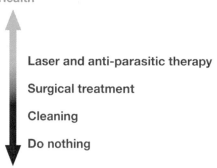

Health
Laser and anti-parasitic therapy
Surgical treatment
Cleaning
Do nothing
Gum Disease

Therapy objective :

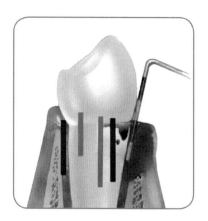

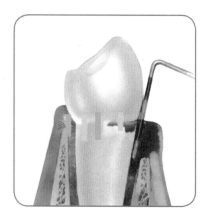

Gradually close periodontal pockets and end bleeding: leading to a healthy mouth and a healthy body.

What Causes Periodontal Disease
And What Is the
Best Way to Treat it?

S ince periodontal disease affects almost 50 percent of the population, we are often asked, "What causes it and what is the best way to treat it?" Periodontal disease is caused by millions of specific aggressive bacteria and parasites that infect the gums and bone around your teeth, and then migrate into your bloodstream to affect your health. Genetics, smoking, diabetes, and the way our teeth fit together can all amplify our reaction to these bacteria.

Identifying and eliminating the animal parasites and other pathogenic bacteria causing the periodontal infection is the best way to cure or control the disease and save your teeth. We were among the first to use the phase contrast microscope and culturing over 30 years ago to identify these bacteria and parasites. (See Four Steps to Eliminate Periodontal Disease on the next page.)

The microscope allows us to actually see the amount and type of disease-causing bacteria and parasites to better diagnose and treat the infection. We have analyzed more than 400,000 microscopic smears and 4,000 cultures, making us among the most experienced in the world in treating the specific infection. The bacteria identified by the microscope, such as spirochetes and motile rods, and animal parasites such as amoeba and trichomonads, have been proven to increase the chance of future bone loss by eight to ten times or more. (See Microscopic Slides of Bacteria Associated With Various Gum Infections on page 17.)

What distinguishes our office is that we identify (See Laboratory Report of a Culture on page 20), and then eliminate, the actual causative bacteria and parasites with lasers, and targeted specific antibiotics and antiseptics. We also adjust the bite to reduce biting stress on the teeth during healing. We regenerate the bone using the laser instead of cutting away the pockets. This is the best way to save your teeth, and protect your health. (See previous page for treatment choices.)

For a a video discussion of this topic, go to mccawley.com/videos
What Causes Periodontal Disease
and What is the Best Way to Treat It?

Four Steps to Eliminate Periodontal Disease

First Step

Provide a bacterial and parasitic diagnosis by using the microscope, clinical signs, and sometimes a culture.

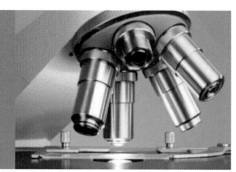

Second Step

Eliminate the infection with the use of scaling, the laser, disinfectant products and specially selected antibiotics based on an individualized microbial diagnosis.

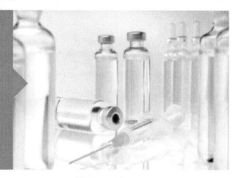

Third Step

Look after your gums and teeth with good plaque control, antiseptics and regular professional maintenance.

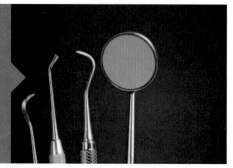

Fourth Step

Avoid reinfection from others, pets, food and water, especially in the Caribbean, and continue bacterial and parasitic control.

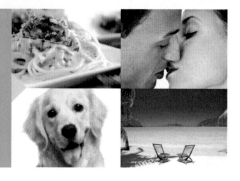

Microscopic Slides of Bacteria Associated With Various Gum Infections And Their Clinical Manifestations

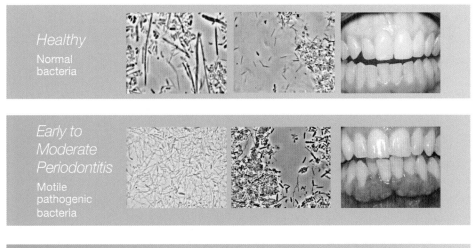

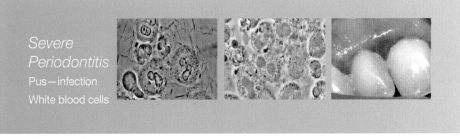

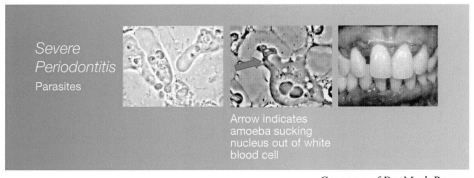

Courtesy of Dr. Mark Bonner

Oral amoebas are one cause of periodontal disease. They also infect the tonsils and lungs. They eat 100 white blood cells in their 21-day life by sucking out the nucleus and releasing toxic enzymes. (See slide of amoeba sucking out white blood cell nucleus immediately above.)

What Questions Should I Ask When Searching for a Periodontist?

T here are seven key questions we advise patients to ask when searching for a periodontist.

1. Does the periodontist treat the actual bacterial cause of periodontal disease, or does the periodontist just cut away at the resultant pockets? (See page 20 for a laboratory report of a culture that identifies the actual cause of periodontal disease, which in turn helps select the appropriate antibiotic to use.)

2. Does the periodontist use the new Simply Perio diagnostic test to identify viruses which occasionally play an important role in the cause of periodontal disease? This test also identifies pseudomonas, an important cause of peri-implantitis. (See Appendix page 76.)

3. When treating periodontal disease, does the periodontist use the state-of-the-art Laser-Assisted New Attachment Procedure (LANAP), which causes minimal discomfort, and stimulates the growth of new bone? (See X-rays on following page.) Does the periodontist also use the new PerioDT solution with desiccation technology that helps kill all the bacteria in the pocket. Or does the periodontist use conventional painful cutting and stitching surgery?

3. For unsightly gum recession, does the periodontist use the much gentler Chao Pinhole gum rejuvenation technique, which uses no scalpels? Or does the periodontist use conventional surgery that creates a painful wound on the roof of the mouth?

4. Is the periodontist very concerned about my comfort? Does the periodontist offer sedation for anxious patients? Or does the periodontist only use local anesthetic shots?

5. Is the periodontal practice privately-owned and operated in the community for many years focusing first on my needs? Or is it a corporately-owned practice managed by businessmen focused on daily production goals, not dentists focused on their patients' best care?

6. Is the periodontist available in one office five days a week to attend to my concerns? Or does the periodontist travel to many different offices, and only visit my dentist's office a couple of days per month?

7. Are the periodontist and staff friendly and personable and have great Google reviews? Do they take the time to listen to my concerns, and then do a comprehensive examination, and tailor a treatment plan specific to my needs and desires?

For a video discussion of this topic, go to mccawley.com/videos
What Questions Should I Ask
When Searching for a Periodontist?

"I recently visited Dr. Tom and Mark McCawley's office to observe and learn new treatment procedures. I cannot thank them enough for sharing their expertise."

Ken Versman, Periodontist
Denver, Colorado

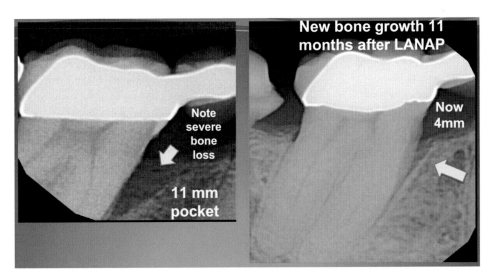

The X-ray on the left shows an unhealthy 11mm pocket with severe bone loss. The X-ray on the right, taken eleven months after LANAP treatment, shows the diseased 11mm pocket has been reduced to a healthy 4mm with new bone growth.

DNA Analysis of Periodontal Pathogens

A 28-year-old female with very high levels of seven periodontal pathogens. This helps explain her very severe periodontal disease at a young age, and select the appropriate antibiotics to treat it.. (See Appendix page 76 for the Simply Perio Test that, for the first time, allows us to test for viruses, which occasionally play an important role in the cause of periodontal disease, and identifies pseudomonas, an important cause of peri-implantitis. See also page 77 for another culture report we sometimes use.)

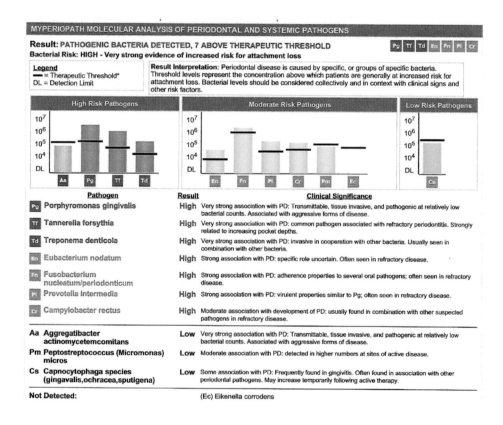

MYPERIOPATH MOLECULAR ANALYSIS OF PERIODONTAL AND SYSTEMIC PATHOGENS

Result: PATHOGENIC BACTERIA DETECTED, 7 ABOVE THERAPEUTIC THRESHOLD
Bacterial Risk: HIGH - Very strong evidence of increased risk for attachment loss

Legend
— = Therapeutic Threshold*
DL = Detection Limit

Result Interpretation: Periodontal disease is caused by specific, or groups of specific bacteria. Threshold levels represent the concentration above which patients are generally at increased risk for attachment loss. Bacterial levels should be considered collectively and in context with clinical signs and other risk factors.

Pathogen	Result	Clinical Significance
Pg Porphyromonas gingivalis	High	Very strong association with PD: Transmittable, tissue invasive, and pathogenic at relatively low bacterial counts. Associated with aggressive forms of disease.
Tf Tannerella forsythia	High	Very strong association with PD: common pathogen associated with refractory periodontitis. Strongly related to increasing pocket depths.
Td Treponema denticola	High	Very strong association with PD: invasive in cooperation with other bacteria. Usually seen in combination with other bacteria.
En Eubacterium nodatum	High	Strong association with PD: specific role uncertain. Often seen in refractory disease.
Fn Fusobacterium nucleatum/periodonticum	High	Strong association with PD: adherence properties to several oral pathogens; often seen in refractory disease.
Pi Prevotella intermedia	High	Strong association with PD: virulent properties similar to Pg; often seen in refractory disease.
Cr Campylobacter rectus	High	Moderate association with development of PD: usually found in combination with other suspected pathogens in refractory disease.
Aa Aggregatibacter actinomycetemcomitans	Low	Very strong association with PD: Transmittable, tissue invasive, and pathogenic at relatively low bacterial counts. Associated with aggressive forms of disease.
Pm Peptostreptococcus (Micromonas) micros	Low	Moderate association with PD: detected in higher numbers at sites of active disease.
Cs Capnocytophaga species (gingavalis,ochracea,sputigena)	Low	Some association with PD: Frequently found in gingivitis. Often found in association with other periodontal pathogens. May increase temporarily following active therapy.

Not Detected: (Ec) Eikenella corrodens

Is Periodontal Disease Transmissible?

Yes, definitely! A three second kiss has been shown to transmit about 40 million saliva bacteria and parasites. If your spouse or anyone you kiss has periodontal disease, it's important they be treated to avoid reinfecting yourself after treatment. Periodontal bacteria, caries bacteria, and parasites can also be transmitted to your children starting at a very young age.

You can also get periodontal disease bacteria and parasites from your dog or cat since they have a high rate of periodontal infection. Those lovable face licks can transmit periodontal disease. Start brushing your pet's teeth at a young age to get them used to it.

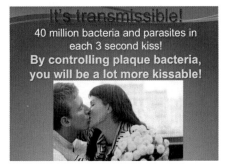

It's transmissible!
40 million bacteria and parasites in each 3 second kiss!
By controlling plaque bacteria, you will be a lot more kissable!

Periodontal bacteria and parasites occur in food and water, especially in the Caribbean. Drink only bottled water, and avoid uncooked food in most developing countries.

Is Periodontal Disease Hereditary?

No, it is a bacterial and protozoan infection transmitted from others. However, an increased susceptibility to this infection can be inherited.

Is Nutrition Important?

Yes. Forty-two percent of people are low in Vitamin D, which promotes bone healing, and 39 percent are low in Vitamin C, which promotes soft tissue healing. We suggest a multi-vitamin as insurance that you are not low in these vitamins critical to healing after periodontal therapy...and to overall health. However, high doses of these vitamins can be detrimental -- more than 2,000 mg of Vitamin C and more than 4,000 IU of Vitamin D. The recommended daily allowance (RDA) of Vitamin C is 80 mg. The RDA for Vitamin D is 600 IU.

In addition to heredity and nutrition, other major risk factors for periodontal disease are smoking and diabetes. However, controlling the bacteria and protozoans causing the infection will prevent periodontal disease, even if you have any of these risk factors.

How Does Gum Disease Affect My Health?

I t is important to diagnose and treat the bacteria causing gum disease, not only to save your teeth, but also to save your life. These bacteria get in the bloodstream and increase the risk of many diseases. (See next page.) Former U.S. Surgeon General, C. Everett Koop has said that "You can't be healthy without good oral health."

Gum disease has been proven to substantially increase the risk of heart disease. A recent American Heart Association study found that it increases the risk of first heart attacks by 28 percent. (See Risk of First Heart Attack Increased by 28 percent by Periodontal Disease on page 24.)

It also increases the risk of Alzheimer's disease. The bacteria that cause gum disease have been found in the brains of 90 percent of Alzheimer's patients. (See Alzheimer's Disease - A Neurospirochetosis on page 25.)

Gum disease has been found to increase the risk of several cancers, including a 55 percent increased risk of pancreatic cancer. **Gum disease has also been shown to increase the risk of death from pneumonia by over three times in patients with compromised immunity. Pneumonia is the primary cause of death in patients with the coronavirus infection.**

In addition, the bacteria from gum disease have been found to increase the risk of diabetes, rheumatoid arthritis, and stroke, making it very important to have gum disease treated to protect your overall health and well-being.

For a a video discussion of this topic, go to mccawley.com/videos
How Does Gum Disease Affect My Health?

"Before seeing Dr. McCawley, my C-reactive protein (CRP)
score was an extremely high 18.5. (The CRP score is a measure
of inflammation and considered a major risk factor for future
heart disease.) After laser periodontal therapy by Dr. McCawley,
my CRP score dropped to 2.7 in the normal range, dramatically
reducing my risk of heart disease. I can't thank him enough!"
Robert Bowen, Wilton Manors, FL

THE FACTS ARE...

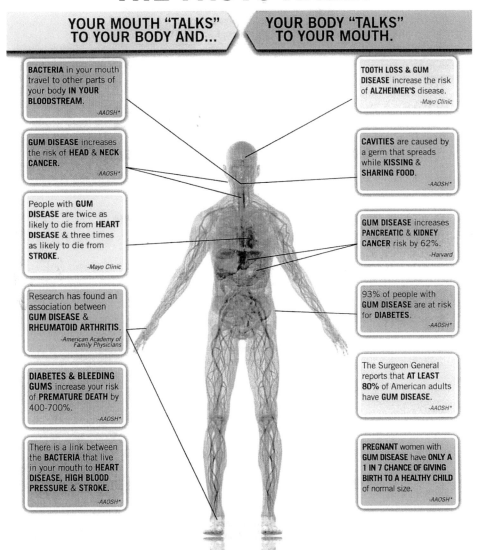

YOUR MOUTH "TALKS" TO YOUR BODY AND...

YOUR BODY "TALKS" TO YOUR MOUTH.

BACTERIA in your mouth travel to other parts of your body **IN YOUR BLOODSTREAM.**
-AAOSH*

GUM DISEASE increases the risk of **HEAD & NECK CANCER.**
-AAOSH*

People with **GUM DISEASE** are twice as likely to die from **HEART DISEASE** & three times as likely to die from **STROKE.**
-Mayo Clinic

Research has found an association between **GUM DISEASE & RHEUMATOID ARTHRITIS.**
-American Academy of Family Physicians

DIABETES & BLEEDING GUMS increase your risk of **PREMATURE DEATH** by 400-700%.
-AAOSH*

There is a link between the **BACTERIA** that live in your mouth to **HEART DISEASE, HIGH BLOOD PRESSURE & STROKE.**
-AAOSH*

TOOTH LOSS & GUM DISEASE increase the risk of **ALZHEIMER'S** disease.
-Mayo Clinic

CAVITIES are caused by a germ that spreads while **KISSING & SHARING FOOD.**
-AAOSH*

GUM DISEASE increases **PANCREATIC & KIDNEY CANCER** risk by 62%.
-Harvard

93% of people with **GUM DISEASE** are at risk for **DIABETES.**
-AAOSH*

The Surgeon General reports that **AT LEAST 80%** of American adults have **GUM DISEASE.**
-AAOSH*

PREGNANT women with **GUM DISEASE** have **ONLY A 1 IN 7 CHANCE OF GIVING BIRTH TO A HEALTHY CHILD** of normal size.
-AAOSH*

COMPLETE HEALTH DENTISTRY™

Designed by Katrina White
*American Academy for Oral Systemic Health

Journal of the American Heart Association February, 2016

The risk of first heart attack was increased by 28 percent in patients with periodontal disease, even after adjusting for confounding factors (smoking, diabetes etc.).

"These findings strengthen the concept that **periodontal disease is causal of heart disease and should be treated,** not only to improve dental health, but also to improve cardiovascular health."

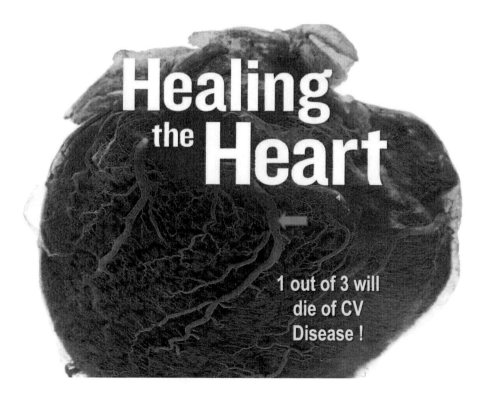

1 out of 3 will die of CV Disease !

Periodontal Spirochetes Found in the Brains of 90 Percent of Alzheimer's Cases

Alzheimer's Disease - a Neurospirochetosis. Analysis of the Evidence Following Koch's and Hill's Criteria

Judith Miklossy
International Alzheimer Research Center, Prevention Alzheimer Foundation
Martigny-Combe, Switzerland

Journal of Neuroinflammation November 2011

Chronic spirochetal infection can cause slowly progressive dementia and brain atrophy. Periodontal disease spirochetes are observed in most patients with periodontal disease.

Spirochetes associated with periodontal disease were observed in the brains of more than 90 percent of Alzheimer's patients.

The analysis of this data showed a probable causal relationship between neurospirochetosis (spirochetes in the brain) and Alzheimer's disease. Once the probability of a causal relationship is established, prompt action is needed.

Spirochetal infection occurs years or decades before the manifestation of dementia. As adequate antibiotic and anti-inflammatory therapies are available, as in syphilis, one might prevent and eradicate dementia.

When Do I Get the Necessary Restorative Dentistry Done?

R estorative dentistry is an important part of overall dental health. Fillings can often be done before periodontal treatment, and active decay should be managed.

Crowns and bridges should usually be completed a few months after periodontal and implant treatment to allow for complete tissue healing.

In addition, your restorative dentist may make an occlusal night guard after your dentistry is done to help stabilize your teeth and reduce tooth grinding at night.

Getting the necessary restorative dentistry done after periodontal and implant treatment is an important part of maintaining your periodontal health, and saving your teeth and implants.

Your restorative dentist also plays an important part in your ongoing periodontal and implant maintenance appointments after active periodontal care and implant treatment. You will often return to that office for this maintenance, or you may alternate this maintenance with your periodontal office every three to six months.

Maintenance is a critical part of keeping your mouth healthy after active treatment to prevent the disease infection from returning.

What Is the **TFBI**$_2$ Home Care Method That Will Help Save My Teeth?

Since almost 50 percent of the population has gum disease, we are often asked, how do I save my teeth and protect my health from gum infection? There are billions of disease-causing bacteria and parasites in the mouth. (See Microscopic Slides of Bacteria Associated With Gum Infections on page 17.) Many live in a sticky plaque which grows on the teeth. It's important to remove this sticky bacterial plaque at least once daily. These bacteria and parasites act like termites to destroy the bone around teeth. We created the acronym **TFBI**$_2$ to help us remember how best to control them. (See illustrations on pages 28 and 29.)

First, scrape the very back of the **T**ongue with a tongue scraper ten to 15 times to remove the bacteria from the tongue. Using a toothbrush to clean the tongue is like using a broom to clean a shag rug. The back of the tongue harbors up to 50 percent of the bacteria that live in the mouth. These bacteria also produce sulphide odors, which are the main source of bad breath.

Second, clean between the teeth with unwaxed **F**loss or other interproximal cleaners, like Proxabrush, Soft-Picks or Stim-U-Dent. Cleaning between the teeth is the most important step since most bacteria and parasites hide between the teeth. Almost all gum disease occurs between the teeth.

Third, **B**rush the teeth with baking soda and/or a one percent hydrogen peroxide solution focusing on the gum line. An electric brush is helpful.

Fourth, **I**rrigate the pockets using a water irrigator or a Sonic Fusion, adding a bacteria- and parasite-killing antiseptic to the water. Controlling oral bacteria and parasites is similar to controlling termites and ants: after kicking over a termite or an ant hill, it is necessary to put some insect killer on it.

Finally, for some patients, apply anti-**I**nfectives between the teeth. (Ask us about the proper irrigants and anti-infectives for your specific bacteria and parasites.)

These simple steps will help save your smile, freshen your breath, prevent disease transmission, and protect your health.

How Often Do I Need to Floss and What is the Best Way to Floss?

Cleaning between your teeth is essential to saving your teeth. Use unwaxed dental floss once each day to remove plaque from the area between the teeth where most disease and mouth odor occurs. If daily flossing is difficult, consider flossing at least twice each week, or using a Proxabrush or Stim-U-Dent plaque remover. Also consider using slicker floss, such as "Glide" or "Listerine/Reach." Ask us for assistance with any problems cleaning between your teeth.

Four-Step Flossing Procedure

1. Hold Floss correctly, wrapped around middle fingers.

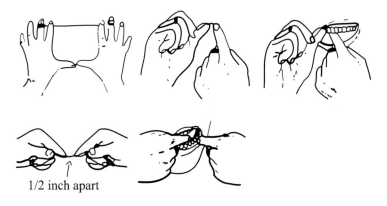

1/2 inch apart

2. Seesaw gently between teeth.
3. Wrap Around Tooth in Tight "C" Shape

4. Floss below gum with three up and down strokes.

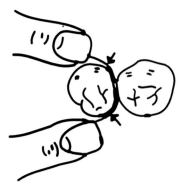

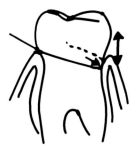

What Is the Best Way To Brush My Teeth?

Develop a system so that all areas are brushed thoroughly each time. **Start on the inside of the lower teeth, brush at the gumline, and use a soft brush for two minutes.** If brushing is difficult, consider using an electric toothbrush. For toothpaste use Arm and Hammer toothpaste which is very low abrasive or brush with 3% hydrogen peroxide diluted in half to 1.5%. It is also available prediluted as Peroxl.

Brushing Guide — Modified Bass Technique

1. Place bristle ends on gums at gum line at a 45 degree angle.

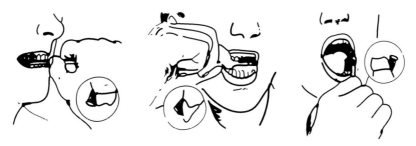

2. Use a short, back and forth, vibrating motion; then two short strokes up or down toward the biting surfaces.

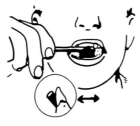

3. Remove plaque from tongue side, use heel of brush in anterior areas.

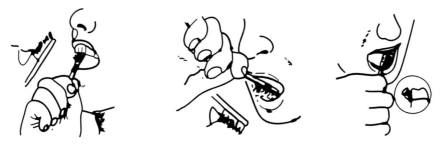

Do I Really Need to Floss?

You are probably wondering whether you really need to floss after the newspaper articles and television reports that there is little research-based evidence demonstrating the efficacy of flossing. We have been following this line of thinking for several years after it began surfacing in the literature, and in Water-Pik and AirFloss ads. We do find both of these products useful, but not as a replacement for cleaning between the teeth first.

Just because there is no long-term study that demonstrates the benefits of flossing, that does not prove the lack of flossing's effectiveness. Because there is so little money to be made from floss, no company will spend millions to run a long-term study with hundreds of participants to test the hypothesis that it works. The bottom line is that lack of high-quality evidence is not proof of lack of effectiveness, especially when there has been so little effort to get "high quality" evidence. We are very wary of these systematic reviews that fail to find a benefit. You do not need to run a study to prove that if you put your hand on a stove, it will get burned.

Actually, you don't need to floss. The old saying, based on decades of dentists' clinical experience, is to "only floss the teeth you want to keep." You can also clean between the teeth with a variety of tools, such as a Proxabrush, Stim-U-Dent plaque remover, or Soft-Picks, but you still need to clean between the teeth.

Think about it. Most periodontal disease and decay occurs between the teeth, and flossing is a great way to reduce both diseases. Nothing else gets this interproximal plaque out as well. The bacteria that cause both diseases live in a gel-like biofilm. This biofilm is similar to the slime that forms on the bottom of a flower vase, or on rocks by the side of a stream. You can't wash this off. It must be disorganized once daily by some mechanical tool.

Yes, we regret to inform you, you really do need to clean between your teeth, notwithstanding the lack of great scientific studies. Just pick your favorite tool.

How Do I Find the Right Laser Periodontist to Treat My Gum Infection?

Patients often wonder how to find the right laser periodontist to treat their periodontal disease. We suggest that you ask five key questions:

1. What is the periodontist's experience with laser periodontal therapy? Our office had the first Nd:YAG laser in the country in 1990. We have successfully treated over 5,000 patients with the laser, making us the most experienced laser clinicians in the world. (See X-rays of our before and after treatment with LANAP on page 32 and at the top of page 33.)

2. Has the periodontist published research on laser periodontal therapy? Since 1992, we have published five research studies, including a groundbreaking study proving that the laser killed all the disease-causing bacteria in the periodontal pocket almost every time. (See McCawley Study on LANAP Killing Bacteria on page 34.) This makes us among the most published researchers on the Nd:YAG laser in the world. (See Published Laser Research Studies by Drs. Tom and Mark McCawley on page 35.)

3. Has the periodontist lectured on laser periodontal therapy at national meetings? We have presented lectures at the American Academy of Dental Research, the American Academy of Periodontology, and the North American Society of Periodontists, as well as at local meetings throughout the country. We have also been featured on Miami Channel 4 television news discussing LANAP treatment.

4. What do other patients and clinicians say about the periodontist? Does the periodontist have 5-star reviews on Google and other sites? Have they received awards from other clinicians for their studies on LANAP? (See the page 33 for a photo of Drs. Mark and Tom McCawley receiving the LANAP Protocol Hero Award for their LANAP studies)

5. Most importantly, is the periodontist and the periodontist's team kind and friendly? Do they take the time to listen to my concerns, and tailor a treatment plan specifically to my needs and desires?

Our LANAP Cases to Save Previously Hopeless Teeth

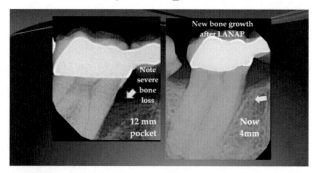

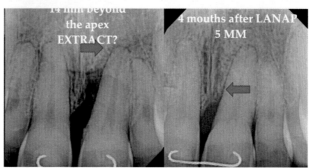

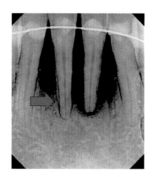 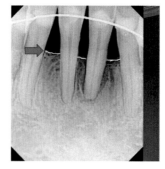

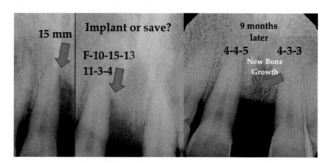

*For a a video discussion of this topic, go to mccawley.com / videos
How Do I Find the Right Laser Periodontist to Treat My Gum Infection?*

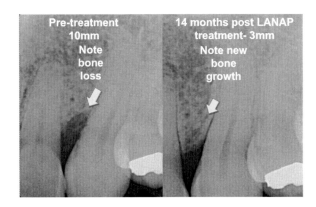

The X-ray on the left shows an unhealthy 10 mm pocket with bone loss. Ten months after LANAP treatment, the X-ray on the right shows the diseased 10 mm pocket has been reduced to a healthy 3 mm sulcus with new bone growth.

*"Dr. McCawley is to Laser Surgery as Picasso is to art."
Don Anthony Tabacco, Hallandale, FL
5 out of 5 stars*

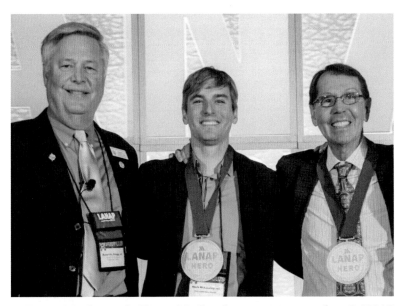

Drs. Mark and Tom McCawley receiving the LANAP Protocol Hero Award for their laser studies. The award was presented by inventor Dr. Robert Gregg (left) at the American Academy of Periodontology 2016 LANAP Study Club meeting.

LANAP Immediate Effects in Vivo On Human Chronic Periodontitis Microbiota

Thomas K. McCawley, Mark N. McCawley
and Thomas E. Rams
Nova Southeastern University, Fort Lauderdale, FL
Temple University, Philadelphia, PA

**Journal of the International Academy
of Periodontology, October 2018**

The LANAP treatment immediately eliminated disease-causing bacteria in 85 percent of deep periodontal pockets. Conventional ultrasonic root cleaning did not remove all disease-causing bacteria in any of six pockets.

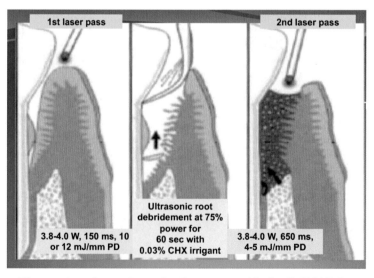

The first illustration shows how the first pass with the LANAP laser removes infected tissue and kills bacteria in the diseased periodontal pocket. The second illustration shows root cleaning with an ultrasonic scaler. The third illustration shows the second pass of the laser seals the pocket with a fibrin blood clot and stimulates new bone regeneration.

Published Laser Research Studies by Drs. Tom McCawley And Mark McCawley

1. Immediate Effects of Nd:YAG Laser Alone on Chronic Periodontitis Microbiota, Thomas McCawley, Mark McCawley and Thomas Rams, Journal of Periodontics and Implant Science, February 2022

2. Immediate effects of Laser-Assisted New Attachment Procedure (LANAP) on Periodontitis Microbiota, Thomas McCawley, Mark McCawley, and Thomas Rams, Journal of the International Academy of Periodontology, October 2018

3. Immediate Effects of Nd:YAG Laser Alone on Chronic Periodontitis Microbiota, Thomas McCawley, Mark McCawley and Thomas Rams, American Association for Dental Research 44th Annual Meeting, Boston, MA, March 13, 2015

4. LANAP Immediate Effects in Vivo on Human Chronic Periodontitis Microbiota, Thomas McCawley, Mark McCawley and Thomas Rams, American Association for Dental Research 43rd Annual Meeting, Charlotte, NC, March 20, 2014

5. Change in Clinical Indices Following Laser or Scalpel Treatment for Periodontitis: A Split-Mouth, Randomized, Multi-Center Trial, David Harris, Thomas McCawley et al, Lasers in Dentistry, February 2014

6. Pulsed Nd:YAG Laser Treatment for Failing Dental Implants Due to Peri-Implantitis, Dawn Nicholson, Thomas McCawley et al, Lasers in Dentistry, February 2014

7. A Preliminary Study on the Effects of the Nd:YAG Laser on Root Surfaces and Subgingival Microflora in Vivo, Charles Cobb, Thomas McCawley and William Killoy, Journal of Periodontology 63:701, 1992

Why Have LANAP/LAPIP Treatment for Gum Disease And Infected Implants?

We are often asked, "What are the advantages of laser treatment with LANAP (Laser-Assisted New Attachment Procedure) over conventional cutting and stitching surgery?" It is an exciting breakthrough in periodontal treatment and one we would want for ourselves if we had periodontal disease. (See LANAP treatment before and after photos below.)

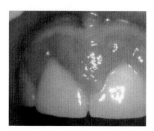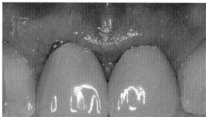

The photo on the left shows severe unsightly gum inflammation and infection before LANAP treatment. The photo on the right shows the inflammation and infection healed after LANAP treatment.

1. It is much less invasive with minimal discomfort after the procedure. You can return to work the next day.

2. It is the only treatment proven to kill all the bacteria in the pockets. We did the study that proved this and presented our findings to the American Academy of Dental Research. Scaling and root planing leaves behind millions of bacteria similar to trying to remove ants from an ant hill with a spoon.

3. LANAP is the only procedure approved by the FDA to regenerate bone around teeth, while cutting and stitching surgery almost always destroys bone. (See FDA Approval for LANAP for Bone Regeneration on page 38.)

4. There is much less gum recession and spacing between the teeth with LANAP, and it can be used to save teeth that previously would be extracted.

Finally, it can even be used to treat infected implants. It is then called LAPIP (Laser-Assisted Peri-Implantitis Procedure). (See LAPIP Case Report Showing Laser Regenerating Bone on Implants on pages 39 and 75.)

For a a video discussion of this topic, go to mccawley.com/videos
Why Have LANAP/LAPIP Treatment for Gum
Disease and Infected Implants?

Steve Brown, D.M.D.
Professor at Temple University, College of Dentistry
Regarding Dr. McCawley's recent LANAP study

"Tom and Mark

Wow!

Beautifully presented. These data offer irrefutable evidence of the positive effects on markedly decreasing pathogenic bacterial load as a consequence of using the laser as defined in the LANAP Protocol.

I do not think I am engaging in hyperbole, when I state that this research is absolutely revolutionary. I am unaware of ANY paper in the literature, which demonstrates the ability to unequivocally eliminate the pathogens most responsible for chronic, progressive periodontal disease.

BRAVISSIMO! THIS WORK HAS BEEN A LONG TIME COMING IN OUR SPECIALTY AND PROFESSION. THAT IT WAS DONE IN A PRIVATE PRACTICE SETTING IS MOST REMARKABLE. THIS ARTICLE WILL ABSOLUTELY BECOME A CLASSIC!

I AM SO PROUD OF YOU GUYS!"

"I was somewhat dubious that this laser treatment of my entire mouth in one visit could be of much help, but my gums had deteriorated to the point that my mouth ached all the time, and my teeth had started to loosen. The results are so much better than I could ever have hoped for! My gums look tight and healthy, they never bleed, and I have new bone and tissue growth. Dr McCawley and his staff are professional, yet friendly and comforting, which was important for me, being somewhat dental phobic. I highly recommend both this practice and this procedure!"

Joyce E., Manchester, New Hampshire
5 out of 5 stars

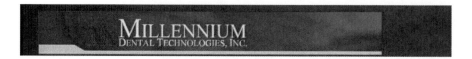

Drs. McCawley: as valued LANAP clinicians, we wanted to make you aware of a historic event. PerioLase MVP-7 has received FDA clearance for **Periodontal regeneration – true regeneration of the attachment apparatus (new cementum, new periodontal ligament, and new alveolar bone) on a previously diseased root surface when used specifically in the LANAP® protocol. (FDA 151763).**

We witness this remarkable breakthrough in regeneration almost every day on patients that we treat with LANAP and LAPIP.

Drs. Tom and Mark McCawley

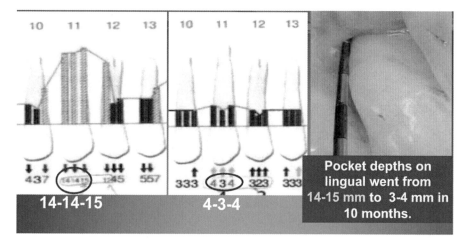

The photograph on the right shows a periodontal probe inserted 3 mm into a healed periodontal sulcus, which the probing chart on the left shows was 14 mm before LANAP treatment. (See before and after X-rays of this tooth below.)

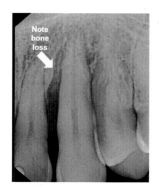
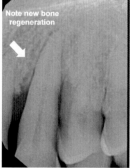

The X-ray on the left shows bone loss prior to treatment with the LANAP procedure. The X-ray on the right shows new bone regeneration ten months after LANAP treatment.

LAPIP Case Study

Courtesy of Thomas K. McCawley, DDS, FACD

LANAP periodontist since 2008, Ft. Lauderdale, FL

PATIENT HISTORY

A 73-year-old female patient was referred for treatment of periodontal disease on teeth and implants. She reported a history of two full-mouth periodontal surgery treatments about 30 and 20 years before. Implants and bridges were placed 13 years before. She was a heavy smoker for about 50 years, but stopped ten years before. She reports that she is in excellent health.

TISSUE CONDITION

Tissue was initially inflamed, and implants and teeth had suppuration. She was very sensitive to probing. Bacterial culturing by the University of Southern California revealed high levels of Porphyromonas gingivalis (3.1%) and enteric rods (2.0%), and moderate levels of Peptostreptococcus micros, Fusobacterium nucleatum and Dialister pneumosintes.

TREATMENT APPROACH

Standard LANAP and LAPIP (peri-implantitis) treatment was performed with the PerioLase MVP-7. Occlusal adjustment was performed, and her general dentist adjusted an occlusal guard which she has worn for 30 years.

RESULTS

Post-op shows tissue is healthy with no sensitivity to probing, bleeding or exudate. Significant new bone regeneration and pocket reduction was noted.

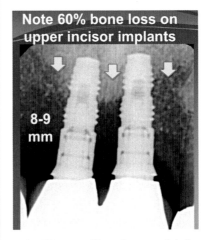

An X-ray of implants which replaced upper incisors infected with peri-implantitis.

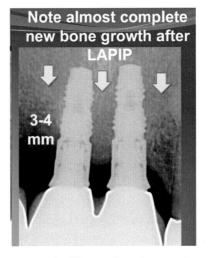

An X-ray showing new bone growth after LAPIP laser treatment.

How Do I Find a Periodontist With the Best Way to Treat My Unsightly Gum Recession?

This is a very good question since there are many possible treatments for gum recession. **First**, does the periodontist primarily use, and is the periodontist trained in, the Chao Pinhole Surgery Technique? This procedure is a much gentler way to cover roots because it avoids a painful wound on the roof of the mouth, uses no scalpels, requires minimal sutures, and causes much less pain. Our office was the first office in South Florida to offer this breakthrough treatment, and one of the first offices in the world to receive Advanced Pinhole Technique Certification by Dr. John Chao, the inventor of the technique.

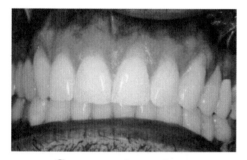
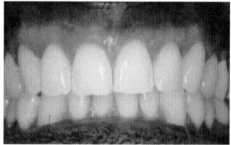

Gum recession prior to Pinhole gum surgery.

Gum recession treated with Pinhole gum surgery.

Second, does the periodontist have credibility in doing this procedure? We were invited by Dr. Chao to lecture at his Advanced Pinhole Technique course in Alhambra, California. We presented our report on a multi-center study, in which our office was one of only three offices in the world invited to participate. We found that in 266 teeth treated with the Pinhole Technique, root coverage averaged 93 per cent. We were also chosen by Dr. Chao, when he visited our office, to do a live video demonstration of his technique, which aired on the Miami Channel 7 television news.

View this television video on our website at mccawley.com or on YouTube

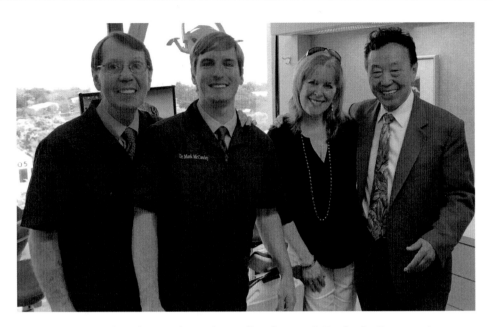

Drs. Tom McCawley and Mark McCawley with Pinhole Surgery inventor Dr. John Chao and Miami Channel 7 television reporter, Leisa Williams, during filming of the Pinhole procedure at our office.

Third, does the periodontist offer other treatments for recession if the Chao procedure is not indicated? We have also pioneered palateless gingival grafting, which avoids taking tissue from the roof of the mouth, is much less invasive, and much more esthetic.

Fourth and finally, is the periodontist concerned about my comfort? Does the periodontist listen to my concerns, and offer sedation if I am anxious about the procedure?

For a a video discussion of this topic, go to mccawley.com/videos
How Do I Find A Periodontist With the
Best Way to Treat My Unsightly Gum Recession?

"Had Pinhole gum surgery done. Amazing results!! There was no pain, just very minor discomfort for a day. Well worth it! Great bedside manner and great staff!" (See before and after photos on the previous page.)

Dino Vannoni, Chicago, IL
5 out of 5 stars

What Causes Root Sensitivity And How Do I Get Rid of It?

O ne of the main causes of root sensitivity we see is eating lots of fruit or drinking fruit juices. Fruit is obviously good for us, but it also causes lots of cavities and root sensitivity. Most fruits are very acidic and contain lots of fructose. The acids in fruits are responsible for much of the root sensitivity that we see. Other acidic causes of sensitivity are vinegar, yogurt, sports and soft drinks, and tea. Check your diet closely for acidic content if you have root sensitivity.

These acids open up tiny tubules in the root and allow cold, hot, or touch stimuli a pathway into the nerve of the tooth causing pain. The pain is usually short lived. If the pain lasts for more than a few seconds, the nerve may be infected and root canal treatment may be indicated.

We recommend minimizing acidic exposure to your roots by drinking acidic drinks through a straw, and eating and swallowing fruits quickly. Rinse with water immediately after ingesting to dilute the acidic effect. Don't brush for at least 30 minutes as the acids soften the roots, making them more susceptible to wear notching. To prevent additional tooth abrasion, start brushing on the inside of the lower teeth with a soft toothbrush, and a small amount of a low abrasive toothpaste, like baking soda or Sensodyne.

The fructose in fruits is closely related to sucrose (sugar). It will cause cavities just like all sugar products, including and especially Altoids, Tic Tacs, and other sugar-containing breath mints.

To help control sensitivity, you can use toothpastes containing potassium nitrate and fluoride, like Sensodyne, and rinse with fluoride rinses, like Act Complete. Over-the-counter Sensi-Strips can be applied daily for ten minutes to block the tubules with oxalate crystals. There are also more potent prescription fluoride pastes available that will protect your roots and reduce cavities. Fluoride varnish can be applied in your dentist's office.

If root sensitivity continues to be a problem, we will sometimes cover the root with the minimally invasive Chao Pinhole Technique, or the sensitive area can be bonded by your dentist.

If I Have Cavities, How Can I Stop More of Them from Occurring?

It is really very simple: reduce the frequency of your sugar intake. However, it's not always so simple to find the source of the sugar, but it is <u>always</u> there.

Tooth decay exploded around the world after sugar from the Caribbean became widely available in the early 1800s. Prior to that, cavities were infrequent.

The problem is that sugar is hidden in many foods. Sugar also occurs as fructose in fruits, which also causes lots of cavities.

Frequency of sugar intake is critical. Every time you put a product which contains sugar or fructose in your mouth, you get a 45-minute acid attack on the tooth, which eventually produces a hole in the tooth – a cavity.

The more often we eat or drink these products, the more often the acid attack occurs. Between-meal snacks, fruits, and drinks with sugar produce this acid attack more frequently each time you ingest them, accelerating your cavities. Sipping these drinks produces constant acid attacks, so it is better to "gulp, don't sip."

Of course, flossing and brushing helps. Using sugar-free products, especially those containing xylitol, will also help. Adding fluoride toothpaste and rinses, such as Act Complete, will make the teeth more resistant to the acid attack, since sugar and fructose are metabolized by bacteria to produce cavity-causing acid.

In addition, a prescription-strength, high fluoride toothpaste like PreviDent 5000 for daily home use, and a high fluoride varnish applied at each maintenance visit will help. A new technology, Durodont Repair Fluoride Plus, can be applied in the office to remineralize incipient decay.

But nothing works like reducing sugar and fructose intake.

How Do I Eliminate Bad Breath?

We all know someone with bad breath because at least 35 percent of the population suffers from bad breath. Unfortunately, most don't know they have it. Even if they do know, they have no idea how to get rid of it. After treating hundreds of patients with bad breath, and also attending the World Congress on Bad Breath in Brussels, Belgium, we suggest six steps to eliminating bad breath.

1. First, determine if you actually have bad breath by asking a significant other or a dental professional. It is not normally possible to determine bad breath on yourself.

2. Eliminate or reduce your intake of odor-causing foods like onions and garlic. These odors come out through the lungs for up to 24 hours after ingestion. These odors can only be masked temporarily by using breath sprays, rinses or sugar-free mints. Bad breath does not come from the stomach, and very rarely from the sinuses.

3. Examine the very back of the throat for tongue coat. There are millions of bacteria on the back of the tongue in this tongue coat. These bacteria produce sulfide odors (the smell of rotten eggs) that are the primary source of most bad breath. We suggest using a tongue scraper to scrape the very back of the tongue 15 times every morning and evening. Using a toothbrush to clean the tongue is like using a broom to clean a shag rug.

4. Get examined and treated if you have gum disease. The pockets under the gum contain millions of odor-causing bacteria.

5. Clean the bacterial plaque from between the teeth with floss or other tools since this is where many bacteria hide. Check the floss for odor: this is an indicator of gum infection and possible bad breath.

6. Finally, be aware that most mouthwashes, mints and gum offer only very temporary help. But mouthwashes which contain zinc, like Smart Mouth, and mouthwashes containing activated chlorine dioxide, like DioxiRinse, offer several hours benefit. Sugar-containing gum and mints, like Altoids, are also a major cause of cavities.

If problems continue, call our office,The McCawley International Bad Breath Institute, for more advanced treatment for your bad breath that is successful almost 100 percent of the time. (See the next page for the Top Ten Myths About the Cause of Bad Breath.)

For a a video discussion of this topic, go to mccawley.com/videos
How Do I Eliminate Bad Breath?

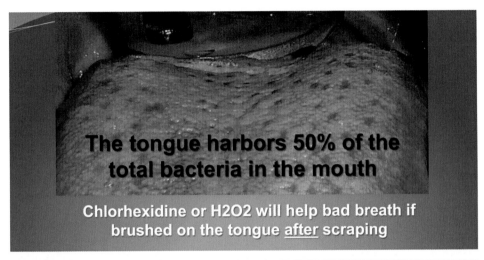

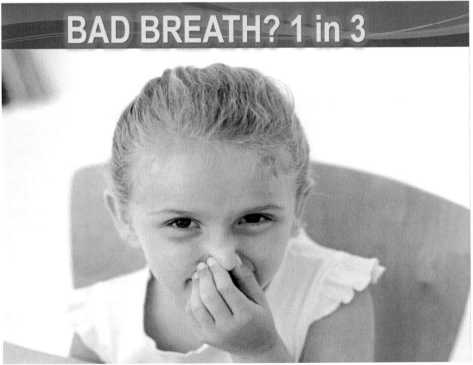

Only your children or grandchildren will tell you!

The Top Ten Myths About the Cause of Bad Breath

1. It comes from the stomach. There are two sphincters that prevent air from coming back up from the stomach, except when you belch or have GERD, so the stomach almost never is the cause of bad breath.

2. Probiotics will help to control my bad breath. No help.

3. It comes from the sinuses. The mucous of sinus infections may occasionally show up in the back of the throat, but is not a cause.

4. It comes from the tonsils. Occasionally people have sioliths on their tonsils. These, when they come loose, can have an odor, but are not a cause of consistent bad breath.

5. The right mouthwash or breath mint will solve my bad breath problem. Mouthwashes and breath mints are, at best, only a temporary cover-up.

6. Antibiotics will treat my bad breath. Occasionally this can be a temporary help, but antibiotics do not penetrate the biofilm causing bad breath, and they don't kill the anaerobic bacteria that don't grow in air.

7. There is no cure for my bad breath odors. The McCawley Breath Center can almost always cure you of these common bad breath malodors.

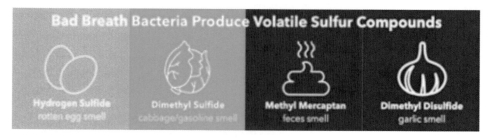

8. It's caused by some medical problem that I have. This can rarely be true, although severe lung, kidney or liver disease can produce an oral odor.

9. Good brushing and flossing will cure my bad breath. Many of the patients that we see with bad breath have excellent oral hygiene.

10. Bad taste indicates bad breath. There is no correlation.

Dental Implants And Implant Loss

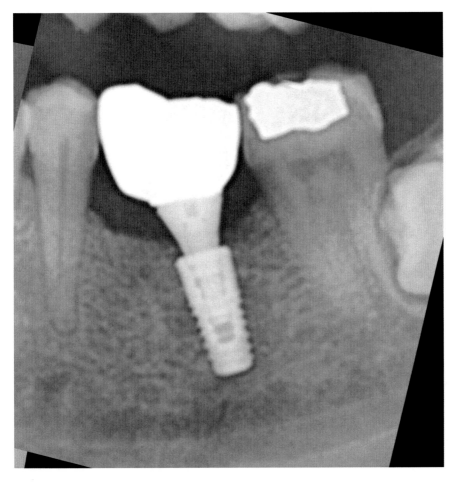

A Dental Implant With a Crown On Top Replacing a Lower Molar

What Are Dental Implants?

I f you are missing teeth or wear dentures, you will be interested in one of the most exciting services in dentistry "osseointegrated" dental implants!

Millions of Americans have one or more missing teeth. Estimates are about 30 million wear full dentures, and that 10 million of them – 33 percent! – cannot wear their dentures comfortably.

Now, with dental implants, you will never again have to worry about loose, embarrassing dentures, or removable bridges or crowns. Some people say that implants feel as much a part of their mouths as their natural teeth once did. (See X-ray on page 47.)

Dental implants are tooth replacements made of a tiny titanium cylinder, which is surgically implanted into your jaw, and then covered with a prosthetic tooth. Through a process called "osseointegration," the artificial root joins directly with your own natural bone, forming a solid anchor which creates comfort, cosmetics and function previously unknown in tooth replacement procedures. Osseointegration represents a significant technological advancement, and is the culmination of many years of research throughout the world.

Anyone healthy enough to have a simple tooth extraction is usually healthy enough to receive an implant. Age is no barrier. The amount of bone available must be adequate to accept an implant. Other conditions in your mouth must be favorable, including the health of the gum tissue.

Dental implants are placed in two steps under local anesthesia. First, the proper type of implant is placed under the gum tissue, and allowed to heal for three to four months while "osseointegration" takes place. In most cases, you can wear a temporary restoration during most of this period, so there is little disruption of business and social activities. The implants are then uncovered from beneath the gum tissue, and the artifical teeth are created and attached to the implants by your restorative dentist

Finally, the comfort and function of permanent teeth are yours!

Our All On 5/6 Cases to Restore Esthetics and Chewing

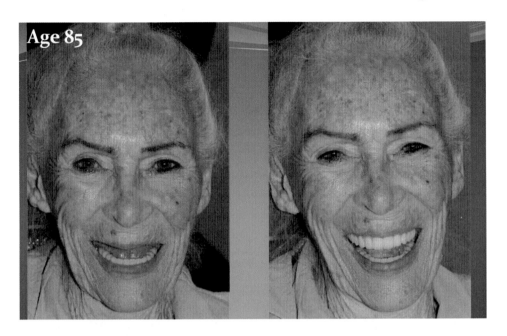

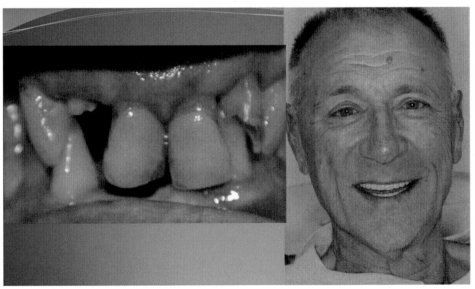

What Questions Should I Ask When Searching for a Dental Implantologist?

W hat are the biggest problems potential patients face when trying to find the right specialist for their dental implants? If you know what questions to ask, it doesn't have to be difficult. We recommend that you ask seven key questions, when searching for a dental implantologist.

1. Does the implantologist have three years of graduate training in placing implants, and teach at a Nova Southeastern College of Dental Medicine implant course? Or did the implantologist learn how to do implants at a weekend course?

2. Does the implantologist use the highest quality, most reliable and most researched implants? Or does the implantologist use cheaper knock-offs?

3. Does the implantologist use low radiation, three-dimensional X-ray scans to plan the implant treatment? Or does the implantologist just use conventional X-rays which often fail to show critical anatomy?

4. Is the implantologist board certified in implant surgery?

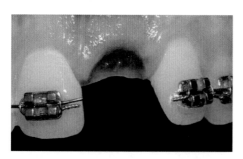

This patient lost an upper central incisor due to trauma.

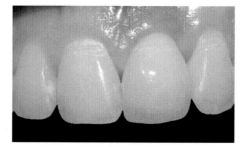

An implant was placed, and restored with a crown to restore the tooth's natural appearance.

5. Is the implantologist very concerned about my comfort? Does the implantologist offer sedation for anxious patients, or only use local anesthetics?

6. Is the implantologist available in the office five days a week to attend to my concerns? Or does the implantologist travel to many different offices and only visit my dental office a couple of days per month?

7. Is the implantologist's practice privately-owned and operated in the community for many years, focusing first on my needs? Or is the implantologist's practice corporately-owned and managed by MBAs from afar, focused on daily production goals?

8. Is the implantologist friendly and personable, and have great Google reviews? Does the implantologist take the time to listen to my concerns, and tailor an implant treatment plan specifically for my needs and desires?

For a video discussion of this topic, go to mccawley.com/videos
What Questions Should I Ask
When Searching for a Dental Implantologist?

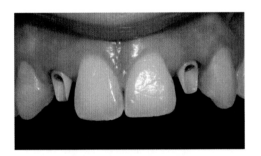 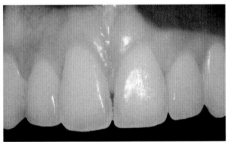

This patient lost both lateral incisors and had implants placed.

The implants were restored with natural looking crowns to restore the natural appearance of the patient's teeth.

Should I Get a Dental Implant Or a Bridge to Replace My Missing Tooth?

In most cases, an implant is preferred because you don't have to cut down the two adjacent teeth to place crowns. Cutting down natural teeth increases their susceptibility to cavities, and root canals are sometimes necessary. Implants don't get cavities and are easier to clean. In some cases, if crowns are already present and need replacement, a bridge is an option. This makes flossing much more difficult, since you must thread under the bridge to clean it.

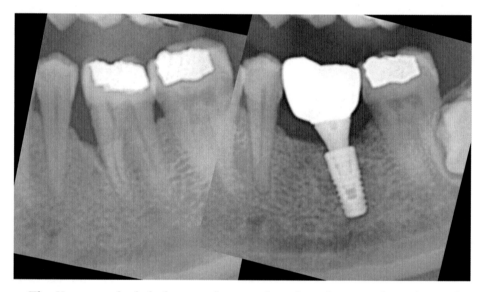

The X-ray on the left shows a fractured tooth with severe bone loss. The tooth was extracted and replaced by an implant and a crown (X-ray on the right) to restore function.

If I Have a Loose Fitting Denture, Can Dental Implants Be Placed To Stabilize It With "All on 4 / Teeth Today?"

Yes, two implants can almost always be placed to stabilize a lower denture. In fact, four or more implants can be placed to produce a strong, firm bite – often the same day – for either upper and/or lower arches. Dr. Mark McCawley uses a specialized, full-arch implant "All on 4" protocol that places five or six implants, and a ceramic bridge, for improved esthetics, and better long-term success. He is board certified in dental implant surgery, and uses only top-of-the-line implants, not generic knockoffs.

Remember that wearing dentures accelerates the bone loss of the jaw and results in the loss of support from your facial muscles, causing you to look older more quickly. Implants can help stop this loss, restore good chewing, and give you a younger appearance in one day.

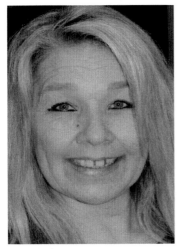

A partially edentulous patient with a hopeless dentition in both the maxillary and mandibular arches.

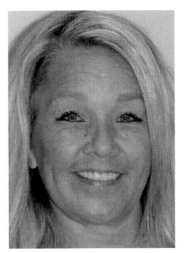

The final restoration of five implants in both arches is both functional and esthetic.

Top Reasons McCawley Periodontics Is The Best Cost to Value for Your Full Arch Teeth Replacement
(Check Google Reviews)

1. We provide a complete implant evaluation, including CT scan and complete periodontal examination for our "Teeth Today" "All on 4" patients to rule out gum disease. We welcome second opinions. Others often provide only a limited examination that misses periodontal infection which can reinfect implants, and overlooks teeth that can be saved.

2. Implants are placed skillfully by a periodontist with extensive experience and with three years of post-graduate training and board certification in dental implant placement, and who teaches others about implants at Nova Southeastern University College of Dental Medicine and national meetings. Others are often trained at weekend courses, and don't teach at universities.

3. We place six implants on every arch when possible, which increases longevity and helps prevent long-term clinical failure. Others usually place only four implants.

4. We only use top-of-the-line, clinically well proven and researched implants. Others often use cheaper knockoffs.

5. We provide much better follow-up care and mainenance in a private practice setting, not in a commercialized corporate clinic. Others rarely follow up or maintain your implants and prosthesis after you are done, which leads to higher failure rates.

6. We also treat your gum infection when present on any remaining teeth and save teeth when possible which greatly reduces the reinfection and failure of your implants. Others in a commercialized corporate clinic needlessly take out teeth that can be saved and don't treat the periodontal infection.

Do Dental Implants Get Periodontal Disease?

Yes, Definitely. It's Called Peri-Implantitis.

Implants are just as susceptible to periodontal disease as teeth, especially if the other teeth present have periodontal disease. The same bacteria that infect teeth and cause periodontal disease also infect implants and cause peri-implantitis. Once periodontal disease starts on implants, bone loss can be more rapid than on teeth. This is because implants, unlike teeth, lack fibers that attach directly to the bone to resist the down-growth of infection. Your dentist or hygienist can detect it with a periodontal probe and X-rays, which may reveal pockets, bleeding, pus and bone loss.

Several studies have found that as many as 56 percent of patients with implants will develop peri-implantitis. A survey of periodontists reported that up to ten percent of implants must be removed because of peri-implantitis.

Once the implant threads are exposed, peri-implantitis is treated the same way as periodontal disease on teeth, including bacteria and parasite control (See The **TFBI**$_2$ on page 27), ultrasonic scaling, and bite adjustment. Special attention is devoted to removing any retained cement on the implant crowns. New laser treatments, such as the Laser-Assisted Peri-Implantitis Procedure (LAPIP), and bone grafting techniques show promise if the bone loss is not too severe.

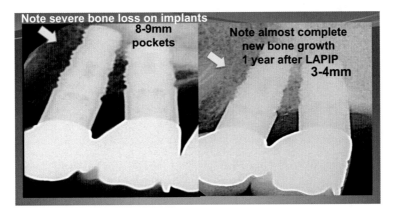

Left: An X-ray of implants infected with peri-implantitis.
Right: An X-ray showing new bone growth after LAPIP laser treatment.

Once Infection Starts on
A Dental Implant,
Can It Be Saved?

Yes. We have pioneered the treatment of infected implants with the Laser-Assisted Peri-Implantitis Procedure (LAPIP), and bacterial analysis to identify and treat the specific infecting bacteria. This procedure has the potential to stop the infection and sometimes regenerate bone. (See LAPIP Case Report Showing Laser Regenerating Bone on Implants on pages 39, 74 and 75.) In more severe cases, bone grafting can be used.

Treatment success on infected implants is variable, but the implants can usually be maintained for years. Severely infected implants may need to be removed. The site can then be bone-grafted, and a new implant can be placed later if desired.

Peri-implantitis can be prevented by good home care, including flossing, brushing, and irrigation, and regular periodontal maintenance visits every three to six months. Early treatment of any bleeding can prevent progression to peri-implantitis.

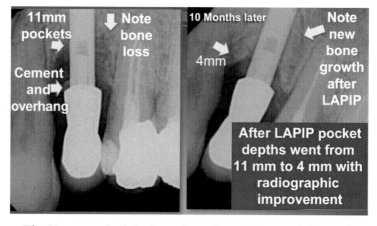

The X-ray on the left shows bone loss all around the implant with diseased 11mm pockets. Ten months following laser treatment, the X-ray on the right shows the pocket depths were reduced from a diseased 11mm to a healthy 4mm, and new bone was regenerated, saving the implant.

If I Get a Toothache, How Can I Determine What is Causing It and How Best to Treat It?

Will I Need a Root Canal?

It depends on the type of pain you are having. If the pain is severe or sharp, keeps you up at night, and is made worse by heat that lasts for 15 seconds or more, it most likely means the nerve of the tooth is dying, and you will need root canal treatment. Other indications that the tooth may need root canal treatment include pain when biting, pain when the apex of the root is palpated, and pain referred back towards the ear. If a root canal has been completed and pain returns, sometimes the root canal can be redone, or surgery can be performed on the infected area. If these treatments are not feasible, the tooth may need to be extracted, and replaced by a bridge or an implant. (See Figures 1 and 2 below.)

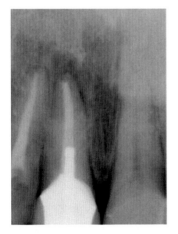

Figure 1. A periapical radiograph shows prior endodontic treatment, which suggests that redoing the root canal would be difficult, and that an immediate dental implant could possibly be placed.

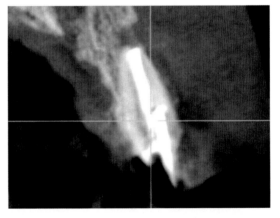

Figure 2. A 3-D X-ray rules out the possibility of redoing the endodontics and placing an immediate implant, due to significant bone loss and infection at the end of the root. An implant can be placed later, after extraction and bone grafting.

Is It a Cracked Tooth?

If the pain is sharp when biting and lasts only a few seconds, you may have a crack in the tooth. If the crack is not too severe and doesn't involve the nerve, the tooth can often be saved with a crown. If the crack involves the nerve, often it can still be saved by a root canal and a crown. Sometimes the gum can be trimmed below the fracture line, and the tooth can still be saved. If the tooth has a large crack or vertical fracture, it will usually have to be extracted and replaced by an implant or bridge. (See Figures 3 and 4 below.)

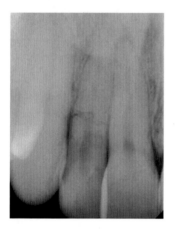

Figure 3. A periapical radiograph reveals a horizontal fracture on the upper right lateral incisor at the level of the crestal bone.

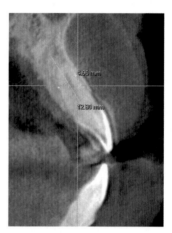

Figure 4. A 3-D X-ray of the fractured tooth reveals good bone thickness, which would allow placement of an immediate implant.

Is It Root Sensitivity?

If the pain is made worse by cold or heat, like hot coffee, but lasts only a few seconds with no pain when biting, this may be due to root sensitivity. Root sensitivity can be treated by desensitizing medications, reducing acids in your diet, or the root can sometimes be covered by the minimally invasive Chao Pinhole Surgical Technique. (See page 40.)

Is It a Gum Problem?

If the pain is dull, more diffuse, less severe, and you can point directly to the site, it is likely a gum abscess in a pocket that can be drained and initially treated with local antibiotics. If the bone loss is not severe, the tooth can usually be saved by periodontal treatment, often with the laser.

How Do I Manage My Fear of Getting Periodontal or Implant Treatment?

You need to find the right sedation specialist. We suggest asking these six questions: First, what is the nature of the periodontist's training. Was the periodontist trained in a three-year, university-based graduate program, with additional training at a leading sedation hospital?

Second, is the periodontist very safety conscious? Is the periodontist trained in Advanced Cardiac Life Support, and is a CPR instructor with the latest hospital grade monitoring equipment?

Third, has the periodontist and the periodontist's team had extensive experience managing anxious patients with sedation? Our doctors and team have safely sedated over 4,000 very anxious patients, helping them to receive the periodontal and implant care that they want and need in a relaxed comfortable way.

Fourth, does the periodontist have the state-of-the-art VeinViewer infrared technology to ensure finding the vein on the first try? (See the next page for a description of the VeinViewer.)

Fifth and most importantly, are the periodontist and the periodontist's team kind and friendly? Do they take the time to listen to my concerns? Do they offer minimally-invasive treatments, using lasers and the Chao Pinhole Surgical Technique, that avoid cutting and stitching, and have minimal post treatment discomfort?

Sixth and finally, does the periodontist use the most reliable and well-researched implants to restore my missing teeth?

For a video discussion of this topic, go to mccawley.com/videos
Sedation Dentistry - How Do I Manage My Fear of Getting
Periodontal or Implant Treatment?

"When you find the right doctor and staff, your problems are over. It is not necessary to endure pain when they know what they are doing."

Gloria Ashley-Emerson, Hollywood, FL

IV Sedation Using the VeinViewer Flex

Many of us have had the painful experience of being poked multiple times when having blood drawn or getting injections. Sometimes it is difficult to locate a vein. Some people have veins that are difficult or nearly impossible to see.

Now there is a technological solution to the problem of hard-to-locate veins. Called the VeinViewer Flex, this hand-held instrument allows dental and medical personnel to easily locate a vein, even in people with very hard-to-locate veins.

Drs. Tom and Mark McCawley now have this technological aid in the office to assist with sedation injections, and to draw blood. The VeinViewer Flex works by using near-infrared light to harmlessly illuminate the soft tissue around the veins to reveal a digital vein map on the surface of the skin. The light is absorbed by blood, but reflected by surrounding tissue. The high definition image is then projected directly onto the skin.

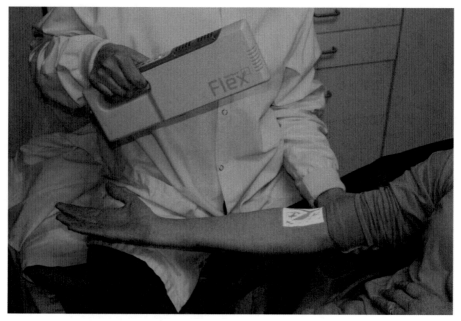

Clinical tests have shown that the VeinViewer Flex improves IV first-stick success by up to 100 percent, thereby reducing discomfort and improving patient satisfaction.

About the Authors

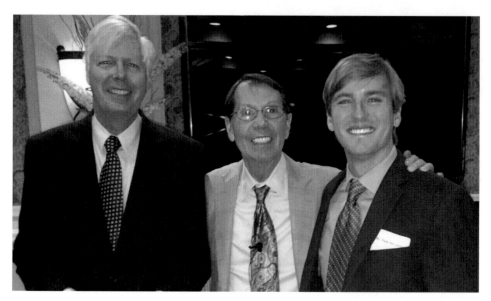

Authors Drs. Tom and Mark McCawley with Dr. Tom Rams, Temple University Professor of Periodontology, after their lecture on their laser studies at a recent American Academy of Periodontology Meeting in San Francisco.

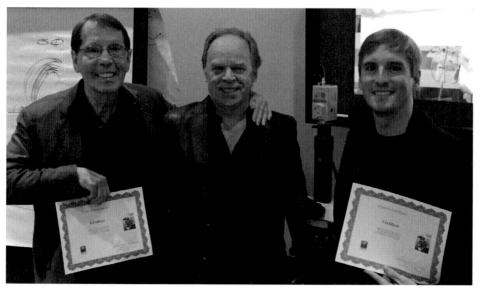

In Montreal, we became the first two US periodontists certified in the Bonner microbiological cure for periodontal disease.

Meet the Authors: Who Are Drs. Tom and Mark McCawley?

Father and son periodontists that live their mission every day "Saving Lives by Saving Smiles." A family practice serving the periodontal and implant needs of Broward County for over 50 years by treating patients like family and giving them the latest leading edge treatments in the most gentle way.

Meet Dr. Tom McCawley, DDS, FACD

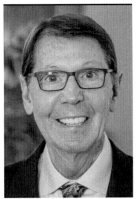

Dr. Tom McCawley has practiced in Fort Lauderdale since 1972. A graduate of the University of Illinois College of Dentistry, Dr. McCawley holds a specialty degree in Periodontics from Boston University School of Graduate Dentistry. From 1969 to 1972, he served in the U.S. Army as Chief of Periodontics at the Baumholder, Germany Dental Center.

In 2020, he was appointed to the Florida State Board of Dentistry to help protect the health and welfare of the public from dental treatments which do not meet the standard of care, and also to help elevate and maintain the professional standards of dentistry in Florida.

He is a Fellow of the prestigious American College of Dentists and, for over 30 years, served as chairman of Clinical Periodontics at the Broward College Dental Research Clinic.

He is past president of the Florida Association of Periodontists and the Broward County Dental Society. He is a member of the Board of Directors of the North American Society of Periodontists and a visiting lecturer at Nova Southeastern University (NSU) College of Dental Medicine since 1997. He recently received an award from the university for more than 20 years of outstanding contributions to the periodontal department.

Dr. McCawley lectures frequently to universities and dental groups throughout the country, and internationally on "Periodontics for the 21st Century – The Latest Advances in Anti-Infective Therapy," microbiology, the use of antibiotics to treat periodontal disease, and laser therapy.

A pioneer in the use of lasers to treat periodontal disease, Dr. McCawley had the first Nd:YAG laser in the country in 1990. He has personally treated over 6,000 patients with laser technology, and lectures frequently on new minimally-invasive, breakthrough laser treatments for periodontal disease. He also pioneered treating the bacterial cause of periodontal disease.

He has presented new groundbreaking research on the laser effects on bacteria to the American Academy of Dental Research, the American Academy of Periodontology, and the North American Society of Periodontists.

Drs. Tom and Mark McCawley recently co-authored two new studies on the Laser-Assisted New Attachment Procedure (LANAP), including a groundbreaking study proving that the laser killed the disease-causing bacteria in infected pockets. (See page 34.) These studies make them among the leading researchers in the world on minimally-invasive laser periodontal treatment. For this pioneering research, Dr. Tom McCawley and Dr. Mark McCawley were awarded the LANAP Protocol Hero Medal at the American Academy of Periodontology 2016 LANAP Study Club meeting. (See page 33.)

After the financial crisis in 2009, he wrote his first book, ***The 4 Simple Secrets to Avoiding Life's Big Financial MESSTAKES.*** In 2020, he published his second book, ***A Blueprint for a Highly Successful Life!,*** a guide to living a highly successful life, finishing well and enjoying the journey.

In addition to this book, Dr. McCawley with his son, Dr. Mark McCawley, has written another book, ***A Clinician's and Patient's Guide: Diagnosing and Treating Oral Diseases and Orofacial Pain, Including Medication and Medical Guidelines.*** All four books are all available on Amazon and on his website, mccawley.com.

Dr. McCawley has also published numerous articles in dental journals and newsletters, and is co-editor of a dental newsletter, ***The PerioDontaLetter,*** which mails to approximately 5,000 dentists in the United States

When he is not practicing or teaching periodontics, Dr. McCawley spends time with his family, plays tennis, exercises, reads, writes, and travels.

> *"How wonderful and compassionate Dr. McCawley is, and what*
> *an excellent doctor. The hundreds of doctors I have seen in my*
> *life, totaled, have not 1/100th the compassion he has."*
> *Christine Jones, Lighthouse Point, FL*

Meet Dr. Mark McCawley, DMD, MS
Board Certified in Periodontics and Dental Implant Surgery

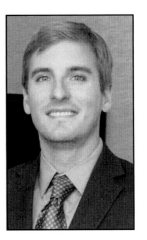

"From father to son, so it goes on."
African Proverb

D r. Mark McCawley is a lifelong resident of Fort Lauderdale. He attended Harbordale Elementary and Pine Crest School, where he was Captain of the cross-country team. He graduated cum laude from Florida State University, and received his D.M.D. degree from Nova Southeastern University College of Dental Medicine. He completed a three-year residency in periodontology and implants and earned a Certificate of Advanced Graduate Study and a Master of Science degree from Nova. He is Board Certified in Periodontics and Dental Implant Surgery, is a Fellow of the prestigious American College of Dentists, and has served on the executive council of the Broward County Dental Society.

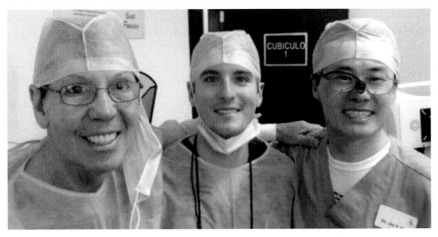

Drs. Tom and Mark McCawley spent four days placing implants in very grateful, underserved patients in Mexico.

He is trained and certified in the Pinhole Surgical Technique, a minimally-invasive treatment for gingival recession, and has appeared on Miami Channel 7 television news with Dr. Chao, the inventor of the technique. Dr. McCawley's was the first office in South Florida to offer this breakthrough treatment, and one of the first offices in the world to receive Advanced Pinhole Certification by Dr. Chao.

Dr. Mark McCawley was invited by Dr. Chao to lecture at his Advanced Pinhole Technique course in Alhambra, California. He presented our report on a multi-center study, in which our office was one of only three offices in the world invited to participate. We found that in 266 teeth treated with the Pinhole Technique, root coverage averaged 93 percent.

He is also trained in the Laser-Assisted New Attachment Procedure (LANAP), and has two published research studies on LANAP. For this research, Dr. Mark McCawley and Dr. Tom McCawley were awarded the LANAP Protocol Hero Medal at the American Academy of Periodontology 2016 LANAP Study Club meeting. (See page 34.) Dr. Mark McCawley has lectured on this research to the American Academy of Dental Research, and to the North American Society of Periodontists.

Dr. Mark McCawley has taken additional advanced training in implant placement, and implant-related bone grafting and sinus surgery, from the Global Dental Implant Academy in California. In addition, he lectured on managing peri-implantitis with the Laser-Assisted Peri-Implantitis Procedure (LAPIP) at the Academy's USA Symposium 2017. He has lectured multiple times to the dental community on his unique modified "All on Four" implant technique (he usually places five implants for better long term success and esthetics) that restores smiles in one day to people with dentures or terminal dentitions.

He is co-author of two books: *A Patient's Guide: Saving Your Teeth, Implants and Your Health,* and *A Clinician's Guide: Diagnosing and Treating Oral Diseases and Orofacial Pain, Including Medications and Medical Guidelines.*

He emphasizes treating the microbiological cause of periodontal disease, not just the resultant pockets. He uses minimally-invasive therapies, such as lasers and Pinhole surgery, in a gentle manner, using sedation where indicated for anxious patients.

In his free time, he likes to play golf, pickleball, travel, and spend time with family and friends.

> *"Many people use the word excellence too freely when describing their services. Yours is the rare case where it actually applies."*
> *Vinnie St. John, Plantation, FL*
> *5 out of 5 stars*

What Makes Our Office Unique?

We are the Most Experienced Laser Periodontists in the World

Drs. Tom and Mark McCawley are leaders in seeking out the latest and most comfortable, minimally-invasive technologies, and state-of-the art anti-microbial therapies to help save teeth and implants. They are known for saving teeth, if at all possible, and placing implants when it is in the patient's best interest. Eliminating periodontal infections not only saves your teeth, but also helps your overall health.

Our office had the first Nd:YAG laser in the country in 1990. In 1992, we published a pioneering study on the powerful effects of the laser on periodontal disease bacteria, leading the way in developing laser periodontal therapy. Since 1990, we have performed over 6,000 laser treatments, making us the most experienced laser clinicians in the world.

In addition to the 1992 study, Drs. Tom and Mark McCawley recently co-authored two new studies on the Laser-Assisted New Attachment Procedure (LANAP), including a groundbreaking study proving that the laser killed the disease-causing bacteria in infected pockets. (See page 34.) These studies make them among the leading researchers in the world on laser gum treatment.

They have presented their research findings and clinical results at prestigious national meetings, including the American Academy of Dental Research, the American Academy of Periodontology, and the North American Society of Periodontists. (See page 35.)

We Treat the Bacterial Cause of Periodontal Disease

Our office pioneered the use of culturing and the microscope to evaluate the cause of periodontal infections. Drs. Tom and Mark McCawley specialize in successfully managing advanced and recurrent periodontal disease by treating the cause, rather than just the effects of, the bacteria and parasites.

Combining microbiology with LANAP allows them to save many teeth that formerly would have been extracted.

We Were the First in South Florida to Provide Chao Pinhole Surgery

Our office was the first periodontal practice in South Florida to provide the revolutionary Chao Pinhole Surgical Technique. Special instruments are inserted through a small pinhole to gently cover unsightly root recession. Pinhole Gum Rejuvenation is a breakthrough for patients and doctors because there are no scalpels, no palatal wound, stitching is minimal, and recovery is faster and pain minimal after treatment. We lectured at Dr. Chao's training course in California, and Dr. Chao was featured with us on Miami Channel 7 television news showing us performing Pinhole surgery.

We Have Extensive Experience in Placing Implants Including "All on Four / Teeth Today" Same Day Full Arch Replacement

Our office has extensive training and experience in placing implants, including a procedure which gives us the ability to quickly replace, in one day, all the teeth in the top or bottom arch of your mouth with a fixed bridge mounted on four or more implants.

We Manage Fear with Sedation for One Visit Treatment

We want to ensure your comfort in our office. In addition to our gentle manner and caring team, we also use conscious sedation to safely deliver care in only one visit for anxious patients. For your comfort, we also use the latest infrared VeinViewer technology to assist in finding the vein the first time to avoid multiple sticks.

If I Have PPO Insurance, And You Are Not on My List, Can I Still Be Treated in Your Office?

Yes, Definitely!
We Treat Many Patients Who Have PPO Plans.

We are an unrestricted provider, which allows us to work with almost all insurance companies. This allows us to provide the best treatment without the restrictions on appropriate care that many plans have.

With PPO plans, you are able to see any periodontist, even periodontists who are not in your network. When you go to someone not on your list, your PPO plan will still cover a portion of your dental fees, often at the same rate as "in network."

Many times we find that your "in network" total expenses are similar to the fees that we charge. At the end of your first examination appointment, you will know the exact fee for your treatment.

If you have PPO insurance, we invite you to come into our office, and we will file your claim for you to confirm all of your benefits.

We also accept most major credit cards, and offer various payment options, including Care Credit to make periodontal health more affordable for you. Please do not hesitate to ask any questions about your benefit plans, our services, or our fees.

What Do Others Say About Drs. Tom and Mark McCawley?

**For more than 1,100 5-star reviews
See Internet – Google, Healthgrades and Yelp.**

**View additional video testimonials under
Reviews and Patient Center-Testimonials at mccawley.com/videos**

"Amazing!! Dr. Thomas McCawley cured my periodontal disease with his laser surgery! He also saved several teeth by using a treatment to regrow bone, making my own teeth permanent rather than having to use implants. He was very good at following up with me for a year, and it was always a very pleasant and motivating session with him. And to top it all off, his office is beautiful, pristine and very professional."

Mary Jo Van Dam, Ft. Lauderdale, FL
5 out of 5 stars

"Dr. Mark McCawley truly put much care towards the health of my gums!! He not only took care of all of my gum work, which was recession of almost all my gums, but was extremely knowledgeable in finding something else wrong. He discovered I had an external root resorption lesion on my lower tooth. He not only saved my gums, but he did the procedure to remove the lesion and saved my tooth!! I'm not the easiest client... I get anxiety and worry over things, especially oral surgery, since I had two previous gum grafts that weren't done to the best of ability. But that all changed when Dr. Mark McCawley took great care of me! I have beautiful new gums now, thanks to his expertise and skills! He and his staff have been most kind to me, and are extremely professional! I feel comfortable and safe with Dr. Mark McCawley. Again, THANK YOU!!! You made a lifelong client!"

Lisa Goldberg, Boca Raton, FL

"I have suffered from gingivitis for a long while. Without effective treatment, the gingivitis became worse, turning into periodontitis. I lost teeth and had bone deterioration. Recently I was fortunate to be cared for by Dr. McCawley and his staff. For treatment, Dr. McCawley used the Laser-Assisted New Attachment Procedure (LANAP). Now I have much healthier teeth and gums. During the entire process of treatment, I had only minimal discomfort. In addition to the procedure going smoothly, the office experience was very pleasant. I would strongly recommend Dr. McCawley for whomever needs periodontal treatment. Laser treatment safely and effectively clears away the bacteria that cause gum disease. With laser there is no need to suture the gum line back in place. Soft tissue is compressed in a way that allows it to naturally reattach to the root surfaces of the teeth. In addition, Dr. McCawley is an inspiring writer. I am grateful to be benefited by reading his book, 'The 4 Simple Secrets to Avoiding Life's Big Financial MESSTAKES.'"

Peter Tsai, Plantation, FL

"My entire experience at Dr. McCawley's office was a very pleasant one. It started with the efficient, friendly and professional staff who took a personal interest in me. I appreciated Dr. McCawley spending time to carefully explain the problem, and exactly what he would do to solve it. The LANAP procedure was painless and I was totally comfortable during the procedure. Dr. McCawley is committed to excellence, and his caring, gentle manner gave me complete confidence in his knowledge and skill."

Sara Tallbacka, Pompano Beach, FL
5 out of 5 stars

"Following a bone marrow transplant for Leukemia in 1985, my gums became severely inflamed. Doctors credit Dr. McCawley's proper protocol in preparing me for the transplant and post transplant care. Thanks to Dr. McCawley and his great team, my teeth and gums have continued to stay in excellent health for over 30 years."

Wayne St. James, Hollywood, FL
Oldest Living Bone Marrow Transplant Survivor in the World
5 out of 5 stars

Pinhole Cases to Manage Unsightly Recession

Case 1

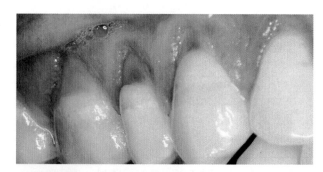

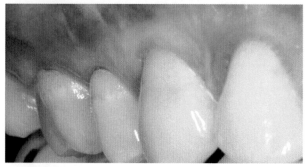

Case 2

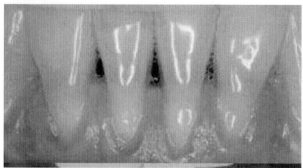

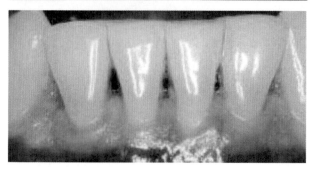

Case 3

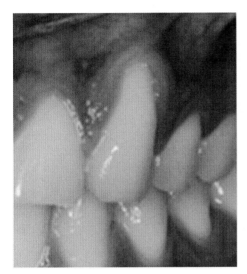 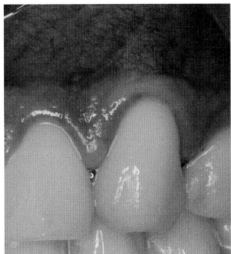

Our LAPIP Cases to Save Previously Hopeless Implants

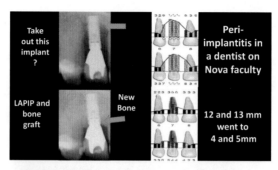

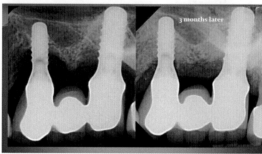

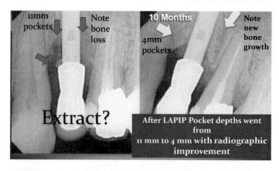

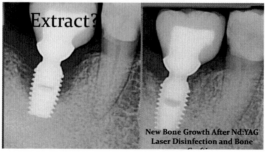

A Previously Hopeless Implant Saved With LAPIP and Bone Grafting

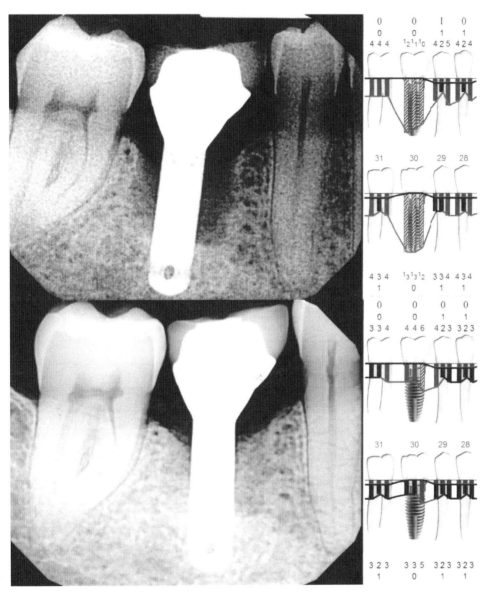

Before and after radiographs and pocket charting of an implant showing complete regeneration of bone after laser treatment (LAPIP) and bone grafting.

Simply Perio Test

The Simply Perio Test for the first time allows us to test for viruses, which occasionally play an important role in the cause of periodontal disease, and also identifies pseudomonas, an important cause of peri-implantitis.

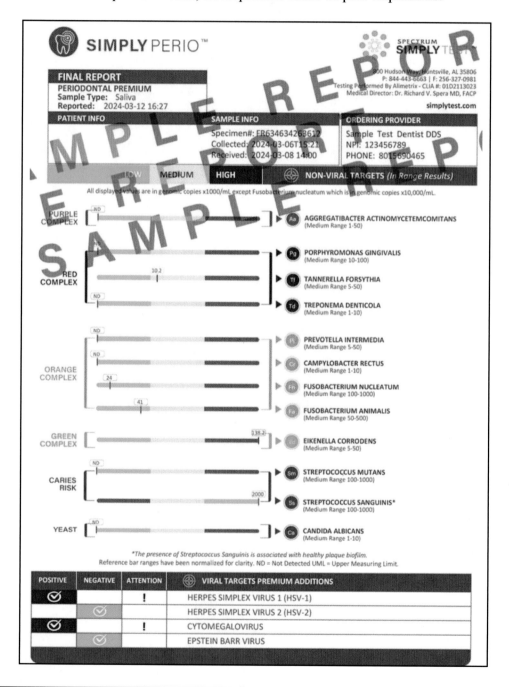

Laboratory Report of a Culture Which Identifies the Actual Bacterial Cause of Periodontal Disease in this Patient And the Appropriate Antibiotics to Use

Laboratory Report Showing Antibiotic Resistance

Putative Periodontal Pathogens Presumptive Identification (critical % threshold level)	% Cultivable Microbiota	Antibiotic Resistance Testing S = 100% in vitro inhibition at threshold value R = resistant			
		Doxycycline (4 jug/ml)	Amoxicillin (8 jug/ml)	Metronidazole (16 jug/ml)	Clindamycin (4 jug/ml)
Aggregatibacter actinomycetemcomitans (0.01%)	0.0				
Red Complex Species:					
Porphyromonas gingivalis (0.1%)	0.0				
Tannerella forsythia (1%)	0.0				
Orange Complex Species:					
Prevotella intermedia (2.5 %)	8.3	R	R	S	R
Fusobacterium nucleatum (10%)	1.7	S	S	S	S
Parvimonas micra (P. micros) (3%)	13.3	S	S	S	S
Campylobacter rectus (2%)	0.8	S	S	S	S
Streptococcus constellatus (2.5%)	20.8	S	S	R	S
Other Opportunistic Species:					
Streptococcus intermedius (5%)	0.0				
Enteric gram negative rods (5%)	33.3	R	R	R	R
Enterococcus faecalis	0.0				
Staphylococcus aureus	0.0				
Candida species (yeast)	0.0				

In this patient's culture, Prevotella intermedia was not sensitive to penicillin because it often produces beta-lactimase which inactivates penicillin. Some P. intermedia species are also resistant to metronidazole necessitating the use of Augmentin which contains clavulanic acid which inhibits beta-lactimase. This patient also had high levels of Enteric gram negative rods which are not sensitive to the common empirical choice of amoxicillin and metronidazole and required the additional use of ciprofloxacin.

Made in the USA
Middletown, DE
29 August 2024

59855966R00044